I0440484

The Hectic Hundreds Chest Workout

Created by Glenn Payne Jr.

NASM, AFAA Certified Trainer

Precision Nutrition Level 1 Coach

Copyright 2022 Glenn Payne Jr. All Rights Reserved.

Workout Program Description

The "Hectic Hundreds Chest Workout" is an intense 10-day workout program designed to target and build strength in the chest muscles. Each day of the program focuses on high-volume training, aiming to push the limits of endurance and muscle fatigue.

The routine consists of chest exercises performed in 100 repetitions, divided into manageable subsets to ensure proper form and intensity.

Throughout the ten days, the intensity gradually increases, challenging the muscles to adapt and grow stronger. Rest periods between sets are kept minimal to maintain a high level of intensity and keep the heart rate elevated, promoting both muscle hypertrophy and cardiovascular endurance.

Participants can expect to experience significant muscle fatigue and soreness during the program. Still, with proper nutrition and recovery, they will also witness noticeable gains in chest strength and size by the end of the 10-day cycle. The "Hectic Hundreds Chest Workout" is ideal for experienced lifters looking to push their limits and break through plateaus in chest development.

Table of Contents

Sample Calendar						
Mon	**Tues**	**Wed**	**Thurs**	**Fri**	**Sat**	**Sun**
Day 1 Bodyweight	**Day 2** Weights	**Day 3** Stability	**Day 4** Fusion 1	**Day 5** Fusion 2	**Rest Day 1**	**Rest Day 2**
Day 6 Bodyweight	**Day 7** Weights	**Day 8** Stability	**Day 9** Fusion 1	**Day 10** Fusion 2	**Rest Day 1**	**Rest Day 2**

Bodyweight Days: Bodyweight Exercises Only

Weights: Dumbbells and Barbells

Plyometrics: Balance Workouts

Fusion 1: Blended Exercises

Fusion 2: Blended Exercises

Disclaimer:

The exercises featured in this workout program are intense, so consult your physician before joining any fitness class or workout hosted by Faster Stronger Wiser Fitness and Glenn Payne Jr.

Faster Stronger Wiser Fitness and Glenn Payne Jr are not responsible for any injuries, sickness, or death from participating in this workout program.

Equipment Needed

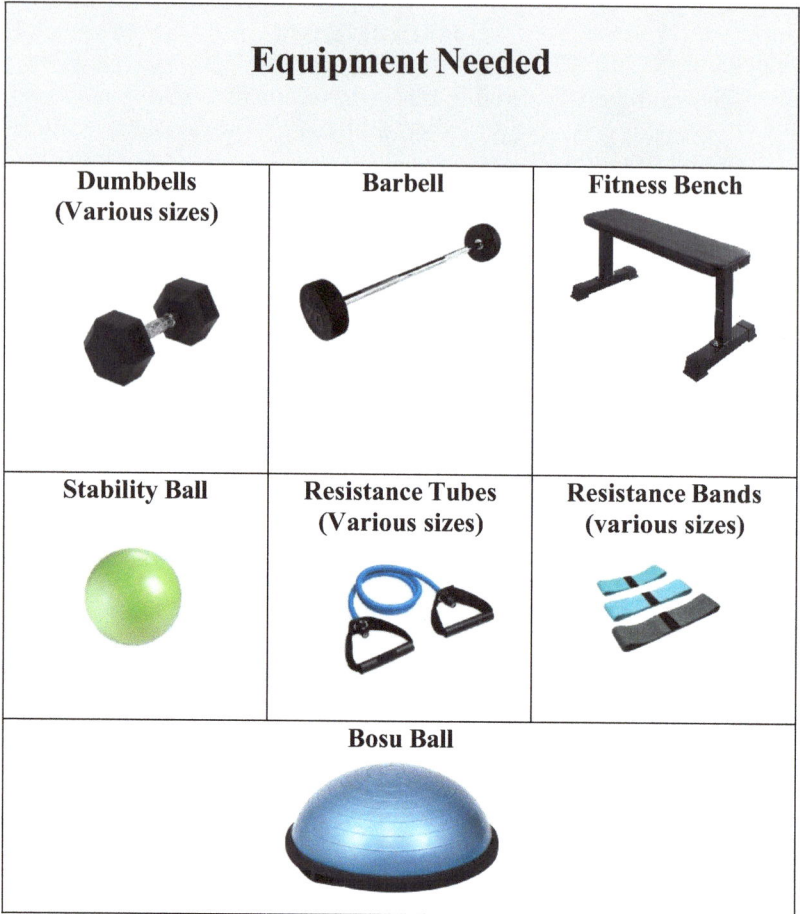

Dumbbells (Various sizes)	Barbell	Fitness Bench
Stability Ball	Resistance Tubes (Various sizes)	Resistance Bands (various sizes)
Bosu Ball		

The Hectic Hundreds Rep System

The Hectic Hundreds Rep System will help you achieve both strength and power in a short amount of time. This process is not based on science but on simple practice. In fitness, we don't see working out as exercise practice; we only see it as necessary to get stronger. When we switch our minds to treat our workouts as practice, we can apply an athlete's mindset to any exercise routine.

For example, a great shooter in basketball takes thousands of shots daily to master the art of shooting a basketball. The same goes for a boxer who practices his punches daily to stay sharp for his fights; if you were to treat exercise like you were practicing for a sport, you would develop a mastery of your body that will make you stronger than you ever thought you could be.

The Hectic Hundreds Rep System operates in three phases, but for this program, you will only utilize two phases.

The Hectic Hundreds Rules

1. Move up weight after 100 reps.
2. Start light.
3. Move up slowly.

Each rep system is progressive and designed to ensure you do not plateau in your workout. A workout plateau is where you stop seeing results in your routine, even though you are training with the same intensity.

These rep systems are primarily designed to be done with weight, but they can also be applied to bodyweight exercises to complete more advanced versions of the exercise, such as a push-up progressed to a clap push-up.

I will review how to track your progress to know when you should re-adjust your goals to ensure you get stronger.

HH Rep System 1: The Hectic Hundreds 4 Quarters

The Hectic Hundreds 4 Quarters is precisely what the rep system's title says. It's four quarters of work, 25 reps for four sets. This rep system is excellent because it lets you quickly get reps using lighter weights. The tempo used in this rep system is 1:1, which means 1 starts the rep, 0 seconds hold, and 1 completes the rep. For example, during a push-up, you would drop down for 1 second, hold for 0 seconds, then push yourself back to the starting point for 1 second. The purpose of this rep system is to flow through each rep while maintaining proper form.

The challenge in this rep system is completing the 25 reps without stopping. This phase is where you develop strength, and it's not about ego lifting. As you transition through this phase, you will gain enough strength to move on to the next training phase.

4 Sets: 25 Reps
Tempo: 1:0: 1

HH Rep System 2: The Hectic Hundreds Double Trouble

This rep system lets you combine high and low repetitions to create a workout that builds strength and power without spending hours in the gym. This was one of my go-to systems in 30-minute sessions because we got to push through 4 to 5 exercises fast while using a decent amount of weight. This rep system is also good for transitioning to higher weights in the middle of a routine since the reps are lower in the last few sets.

This rep system consists of 8 sets, with the reps dropping by five after every two sets. The tempo used for this rep system will be a 1:2:1 cadence. The 2-second pause in the middle will allow more strength and stability to develop throughout the exercise.

Set 1: 20 Reps	**Set 1: 10 Reps**
Set 2: 20 Reps	**Set 2: 10 Reps**
Set 3: 15 Reps	**Set 3: 5 Reps**
Set 4: 15 Reps	**Set 4: 5 Reps**
Tempo: 1:2: 1	

Week One

The first week of this program uses the Hectic Hundreds 4 Quarters Rep System. All weight used this week should be lower because the time under tension or you will spend lifting the weight will be longer.

Day 1: Bodyweight

This day focuses on bodyweight exercises and targets all areas of the chest from the upper to the lower.

Hero Training Warmup (Complete in a circuit)			
Exercise	**Sets**	**Reps**	**Tempo**
1 Shoulder Tap to Superman	2	10	1:1:1
2 Split Stance Walk Out Combo	2	10	1:1:1

Workout (Complete in a circuit)				
Exercise	**Sets**	**Reps**	**Tempo**	**Weight**
1 Push Ups	4	25	1:0:1	Body Weight
2 Dips	4	25 Both Sides	1:0:1	Body Weight
3 Incline Push Ups	4	25 Both Sides	1:0:1	Body Weight
4 Decline Push Ups	4	25 Both Sides	1:0:1	Body Weight
5 Diamond Push Ups	4	25	1:0:1	Body Weight

Hero Training Cool Down			
Exercise	**Sets**	**Reps**	**Tempo**
1 Split Stance Walk Out Combo	1	10	1:1:1

Day 2: Weights

This day focuses on weighted exercises only, and it targets single-arm and double-arm exercises.

	Hero Training Warmup (Complete in a circuit)			
	Exercise	**Sets**	**Reps**	**Tempo**
1	Shoulder Tap to Superman	2	10	1:1:1
2	Split Stance Walk Out Combo	2	10	1:1:1

	Workout (Complete in a circuit)				
	Exercise	**Sets**	**Reps**	**Tempo**	**Weight**
1	Dumbbell Chest Press	4	25	1:0:1	Moderately Heavy
2	Single Arm Dumbbell Chest Press	4	25 Both Sides	1:0:1	Moderately Heavy
3	Barbell Bench Press	4	25	1:0:1	Heavy Weight
4	Alternating Barbell Press	4	25 Both Sides	1:0:1	Moderately Weight
5	Dumbbell Triceps Press on Stability Ball	4	25	1:0:1	Moderately Weight

	Hero Training Cool Down			
	Exercise	**Sets**	**Reps**	**Tempo**
1	Split Stance Walk Out Combo	1	10	1:1:1

Day 3: Stability

This day focuses on plyometrics exercises only, and it targets all explosive exercises.

Hero Training Warmup (Complete in a circuit)			
Exercise	**Sets**	**Reps**	**Tempo**
1 Shoulder Tap to Superman	2	10	1:1:1
2 Split Stance Walk Out Combo	2	10	1:1:1

Workout (Complete in a circuit)				
Exercise	**Sets**	**Reps**	**Tempo**	**Weight**
1 Clap Push Ups	4	25 Both Sides	1:0:1	Body Weight
2 Superman Push Ups	4	25	1:0:1	Body Weight
3 Plank Hops	4	25	1:0:1	Body Weight
4 Plank Ups	4	25 Both Sides	1:0:1	Body Weight
5 Plank Push Ups	4	25 Both Sides	1:0:1	Body Weight

Hero Training Cool Down			
Exercise	**Sets**	**Reps**	**Tempo**
1 Split Stance Walk Out Combo	1	10	1:1:1

Day 4: Fusion 1

This day focuses on combining weight and stability exercises.

Hero Training Warmup (Complete in a circuit)			
Exercise	Sets	Reps	Tempo
1	Shoulder Tap to Superman	2	10	1:1:1
2	Split Stance Walk Out Combo	2	10	1:1:1

Workout (Complete in a circuit)				
Exercise	Sets	Reps	Tempo	Weight
1	Stability Ball Push-ups	4	25	1:0:1	Body Weight
2	Resistance Tube Chest Press on Stability Ball	4	25	1:0:1	Body Weight
3	Dumbbell Single Arm Chest Press on Stability Ball	4	25	1:0:1	Moderately Weight
4	Dumbbell Triceps Press on Stability Ball	4	25	1:0:1	Moderately Weight
5	Resistance Band Pec Fly on Stability Ball	4	25	1:0:1	Body Weight

Hero Training Cool Down			
Exercise	Sets	Reps	Tempo
1	Split Stance Walk Out Combo	1	10	1:1:1

Day 5: Fusion 2

This day focuses on combining weight and stability exercises again.

Hero Training Warmup (Complete in a circuit)			
Exercise	**Sets**	**Reps**	**Tempo**
1	Shoulder Tap to Superman	2	10	1:1:1
2	Split Stance Walk Out Combo	2	10	1:1:1

Workout (Complete in a circuit)				
Exercise	**Sets**	**Reps**	**Tempo**	**Weight**
1	Push Ups	4	25	1:0:1	Body Weight
2	Clap Push Ups	4	25	1:0:1	Body Weight
3	Dumbbell Chest Press	4	25	1:0:1	Moderately Heavy
4	Barbell Bench Press	4	25 Both Sides	1:0:1	Heavy Weight
5	Stability Ball Push-ups	4	25 Both Sides	1:0:1	Moderately Heavy

Hero Training Cool Down			
Exercise	**Sets**	**Reps**	**Tempo**
1	Split Stance Walk Out Combo	1	10	1:1:1

Week Two

The second week of this program uses the Hectic Hundreds Double Trouble System. All weights used this week can be higher because the time under tension or you will spend lifting the weight will be shorter.

Day 6: Bodyweight

This day repeats Day 1 with the Double Trouble Rep System.

Hero Training Warmup (Complete in a circuit)				
	Exercise	**Sets**	**Reps**	**Tempo**
1	Shoulder Tap to Superman	2	10	1:1:1
2	Split Stance Walk Out Combo	2	10	1:1:1

Workout (Complete in a circuit)				
	Exercise	**Sets & Reps**	**Tempo**	**Weight**
1	Push Ups	2 Sets of 20 Reps	1:0:1	Body Weight
2	Dips	2 Sets of 15 Reps	1:0:1	Body Weight
3	Incline Push Ups		1:0:1	Body Weight
4	Decline Push Ups	2 Sets of 10 Reps	1:0:1	Body Weight
5	Diamond Push Ups	2 Sets of 5 Reps	1:0:1	Body Weight

Hero Training Cool Down				
	Exercise	**Sets**	**Reps**	**Tempo**
1	Split Stance Walk Out Combo	1	10	1:1:1

Day 7: Weights

This day repeats Day 2 with the Double Trouble Rep System.

Hero Training Warmup (Complete in a circuit)				
	Exercise	**Sets**	**Reps**	**Tempo**
1	Shoulder Tap to Superman	2	10	1:1:1
2	Split Stance Walk Out Combo	2	10	1:1:1

Workout (Complete in a circuit)				
	Exercise	**Sets & Reps**	**Tempo**	**Weight**
1	Dumbbell Chest Press	2 Sets of 20 Reps	1:0:1	Moderately Heavy
2	Single Arm Dumbbell Chest Press Both Sides	2 Sets of 15 Reps	1:0:1	Moderately Heavy
3	Barbell Bench Press	2 Sets of 10 Reps	1:0:1	Heavy Weight
4	Alternating Barbell Press Both Sides	2 Sets of 5 Reps	1:0:1	Moderately Weight
5	Dumbbell Triceps Press on Stability Ball		1:0:1	Moderately Weight

Hero Training Cool Down				
	Exercise	**Sets**	**Reps**	**Tempo**
1	Split Stance Walk Out Combo	1	10	1:1:1

Day 8: Stability

This day repeats Day 3 with the Double Trouble Rep System.

Hero Training Warmup (Complete in a circuit)				
	Exercise	**Sets**	**Reps**	**Tempo**
1	Shoulder Tap to Superman	2	10	1:1:1
2	Split Stance Walk Out Combo	2	10	1:1:1

Workout (Complete in a circuit)				
	Exercise	**Sets & Reps**	**Tempo**	**Weight**
1	Clap Push Ups	2 Sets of 20 Reps	1:0:1	Body Weight
2	Superman Push Ups	2 Sets of 15 Reps	1:0:1	Body Weight
3	Plank Hops	2 Sets of 10 Reps	1:0:1	Body Weight
4	Plank Ups	2 Sets of 5 Reps	1:0:1	Body Weight
5	Plank Push Ups		1:0:1	Body Weight

Hero Training Cool Down				
	Exercise	**Sets**	**Reps**	**Tempo**
1	Split Stance Walk Out Combo	1	10	1:1:1

Day 9: Fusion 1

This day repeats Day 4 with the Double Trouble Rep System.

	Hero Training Warmup (Complete in a circuit)			
	Exercise	**Sets**	**Reps**	**Tempo**
1	Shoulder Tap to Superman	2	10	1:1:1
2	Split Stance Walk Out Combo	2	10	1:1:1

	Workout (Complete in a circuit)			
	Exercise	**Sets & Reps**	**Tempo**	**Weight**
1	Stability Ball Push-ups	2 Sets of 20 Reps	1:0:1	Body Weight
2	Resistance Tube Chest Press on Stability Ball	2 Sets of 15 Reps	1:0:1	Body Weight
3	Dumbbell Single Arm Chest Press on Stability Ball	2 Sets of 10 Reps	1:0:1	Moderately Weight
4	Dumbbell Triceps Press on Stability Ball	2 Sets of 5 Reps	1:0:1	Moderately Weight
5	Resistance Band Pec Fly on Stability Ball		1:0:1	Body Weight

	Hero Training Cool Down			
	Exercise	**Sets**	**Reps**	**Tempo**
1	Split Stance Walk Out Combo	1	10	1:1:1

Day 10: Fusion 2

This day repeats Day 5 with the Double Trouble Rep System.

Hero Training Warmup (Complete in a circuit)			
Exercise	**Sets**	**Reps**	**Tempo**
1	Shoulder Tap to Superman	2	10	1:1:1
2	Split Stance Walk Out Combo	2	10	1:1:1

Workout (Complete in a circuit)			
Exercise	**Sets & Reps**	**Tempo**	**Weight**
1 Push Ups	2 Sets of 20 Reps	1:0:1	Body Weight
2 Clap Push Ups	2 Sets of 15 Reps	1:0:1	Body Weight
3 Dumbbell Chest Press	2 Sets of 10 Reps	1:0:1	Moderately Heavy
4 Barbell Bench Press	2 Sets of 5 Reps	1:0:1	Heavy Weight
5 Stability Ball Push-ups		1:0:1	Moderately Heavy

Hero Training Cool Down			
Exercise	**Sets**	**Reps**	**Tempo**
1	Split Stance Walk Out Combo	1	10	1:1:1

Hectic Hundreds Chest Workout Exercise List

Shoulder Taps to Superman
Start in a plank position with your hands under your shoulders and your feet hip-width apart. Tap your shoulders with each hand, then lower yourself to the ground. Next, extend your arms in front of your body and lift your chest, arms, and legs off the ground as if you were flying. Return to the plank position.

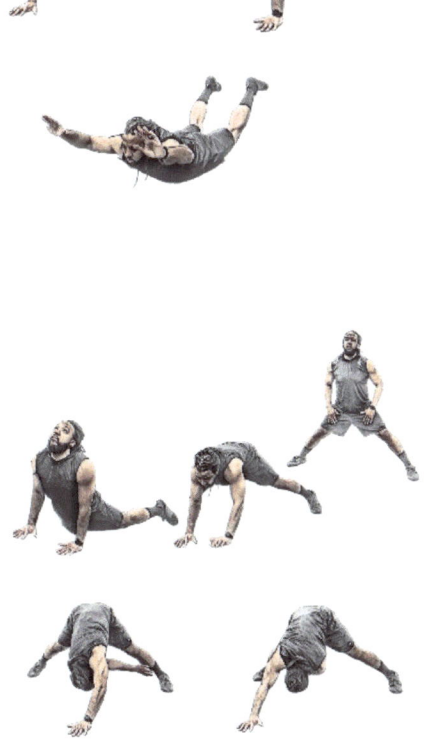

Split Stance Walk Out Combo
Start with your feet in a split stance. Next, bend forward until your hands touch the ground. Walk your hands out until you are in a cobra stretch.
Focus on pressing your hips into the ground for 3 seconds. Next, release the stretch and touch your toes, going right hand to left toe and left hand to right toe. Return to the starting point.

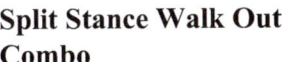

Push Ups

Begin by lying face down on the floor. Place your hands flat on the floor, slightly wider than shoulder-width apart. Your fingers should be pointing forward or slightly turned out.

Keep your body in a straight line from your head to your heels. Engage your core muscles to stabilize your spine. Lower your body towards the floor by bending your elbows. Keep your elbows close to your body, not flared out to the sides. Lower yourself until your chest almost touches the floor or your upper arms parallel the ground. Maintain a controlled movement throughout this phase. Push through your palms to straighten your arms and return to the starting position. Exhale as you push up. Keep your body straight throughout the movement, avoiding sagging or arching your back.

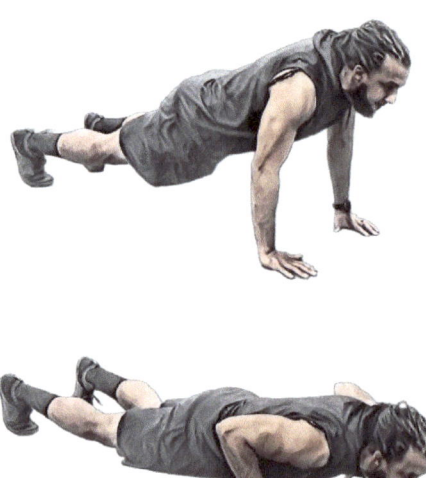

Dips

Position a bench behind you and stand facing away from it. Place your hands on the edge of the bench, slightly wider than shoulder-width apart, with your fingers gripping the edge.

Extend your legs before you, keeping your heels on the ground and your knees slightly bent.

Lower your body by bending your elbows, allowing your upper arms to move parallel to the floor. Keep your torso upright, and avoid leaning too far forward.

Lower yourself until your upper arms are parallel to the floor or slightly below, but avoid letting your shoulders roll forward.

Push yourself back up to the starting position by straightening your arms and exhaling as you press.

Keep your elbows slightly bent at the top to maintain muscle tension.

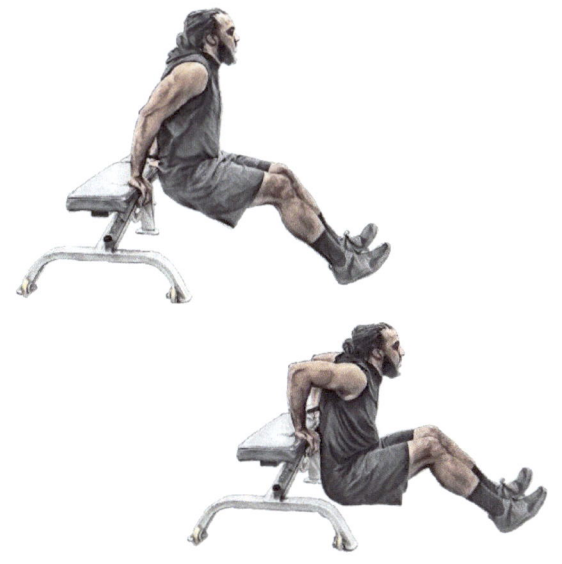

Incline Push Ups

Find an elevated surface: Look for a sturdy surface that is elevated off the ground, such as a bench, a sturdy table, or a raised platform. Make sure the surface is stable and can support your body weight.

Place your hands on the elevated surface slightly wider than shoulder-width apart. Your fingers should be pointing forward or slightly turned outward.

Extend your legs behind you and balance on the balls of your feet. Your body should form a straight line from your head to your heels, engaging your core muscles to maintain stability.

Bend your elbows and lower your chest towards the elevated surface while keeping your body straight. Lower yourself until your chest almost touches the surface.

Press through your palms and straighten your arms to push yourself back to the starting position. Keep your core engaged and your body straighten throughout the movement.

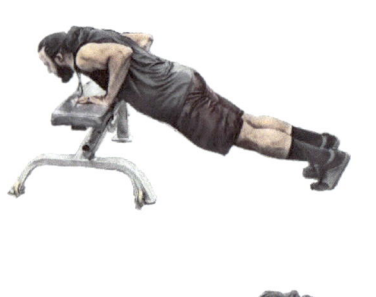

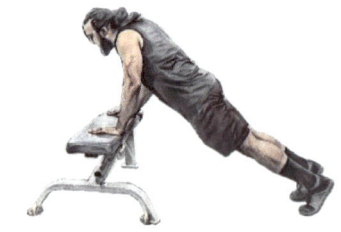

Decline Push Ups

Find a sturdy bench or elevated surface that is about knee height. Make sure it can support your weight without slipping. Assume a standard push-up position with your hands slightly wider than shoulder-width apart on the floor, directly under your shoulders. Place your feet on the bench behind you, with your toes pointing down and your body forming a straight line from head to heels. Engage your core muscles to keep your body stable and prevent your hips from sagging or rising too high. Lower your chest towards the floor by bending your elbows, keeping them close to your body at a 45-degree angle. Lower yourself until your chest almost touches the floor or you reach a comfortable range of motion. Push through your palms to straighten your arms and return to the starting position, keeping your body in a straight line throughout the movement.

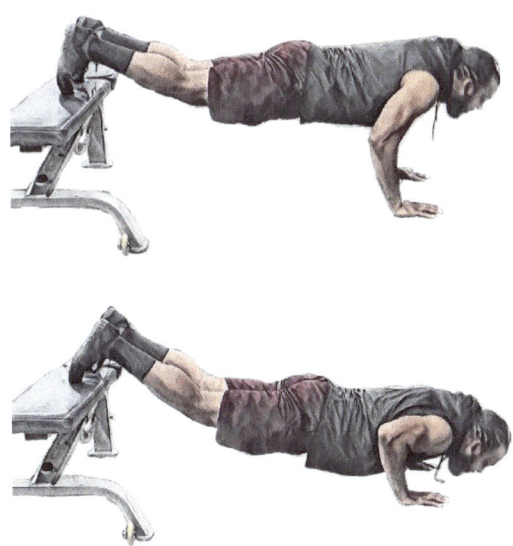

Diamond Push Ups

Start in a high plank position with your hands directly beneath your shoulders and your body forming a straight line from your head to your heels.

Bring your hands together to form a diamond shape by touching your thumbs and index fingers. Your hands should be positioned directly under your chest.

Engage your core and lower your body towards the ground by bending your elbows, keeping them close to your sides. Aim to lower your chest until it nearly touches the backs of your hands.

Pause briefly at the bottom of the movement, then press through your palms to push yourself back up to the starting position, fully extending your arms without locking your elbows.

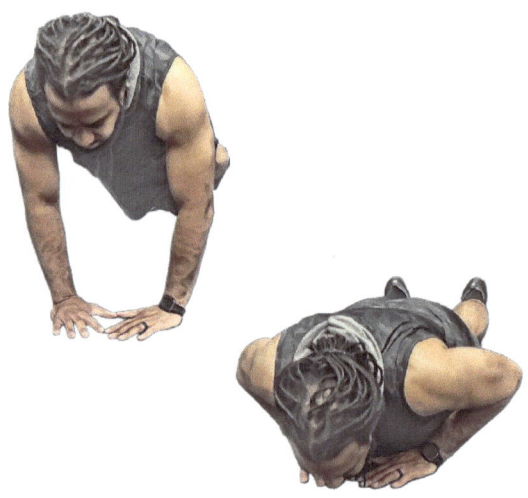

Dumbbell Chest Press

Begin by lying on a flat bench with a dumbbell in each hand. Your feet should be firmly planted on the ground, and your back should be flat against the bench.

Hold the dumbbells directly above your chest, with your palms facing forward and arms fully extended. Your elbows should be slightly bent but not locked.

Inhale and slowly lower the dumbbells out to the sides until your elbows are at a 90-degree angle, or slightly below if comfortable, keeping your wrists firm and aligned with your elbows.

Exhale and push the dumbbells back up to the starting position by straightening your arms while keeping your back and head in contact with the bench. Focus on engaging your chest muscles throughout the movement.

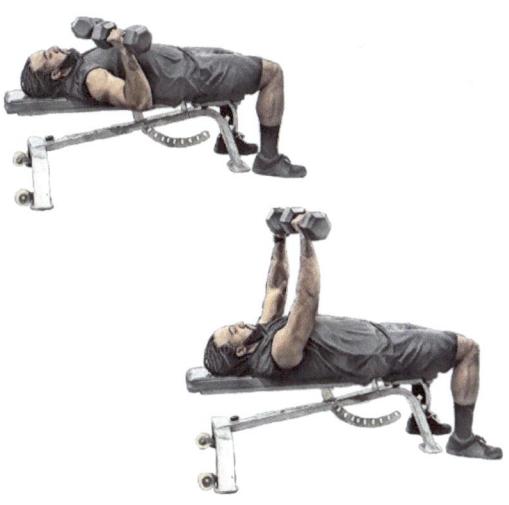

Single Arm Dumbbell Chest Press

Lie on a flat bench holding a dumbbell in one hand with your arm extended towards the ceiling, perpendicular to your body. - Keep your feet flat on the ground for stability.

Lower the dumbbell slowly towards your chest while maintaining control and slightly bending your elbow.

-Press the weight back up to the starting position, fully extending your arm.

Repeat for the desired number of repetitions before switching arms.

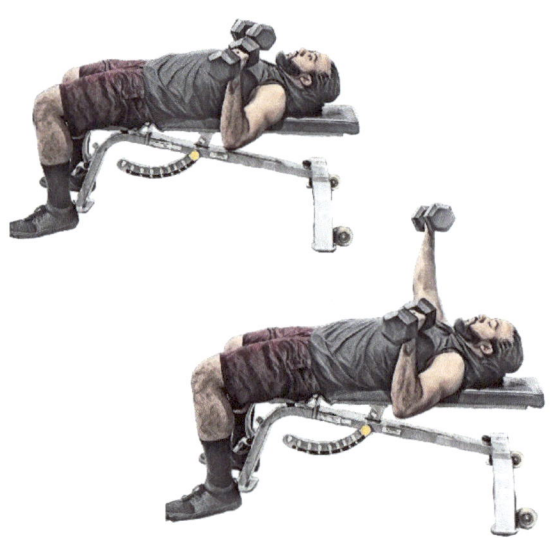

Dumbbell Triceps Press on Stability Ball

Sit on a stability ball with your feet planted firmly on the ground, hip-width apart. Hold a dumbbell in each hand and let your arms hang down by your sides.

Walk your feet forward and roll your body down on the ball until your upper back and head are supported by the ball and your hips are parallel to the floor. Your knees should be bent at a 90-degree angle.

Engage your core muscles to stabilize your body on the ball. Keep your elbows close to your head and your palms facing forward, with the dumbbells above your chest.

Inhale as you bend your elbows and lower the dumbbells towards your shoulders, keeping your upper arms stationary and parallel to the floor. Exhale as you extend your elbows and press the dumbbells back up to the starting position, fully extending your arms without locking your elbows.

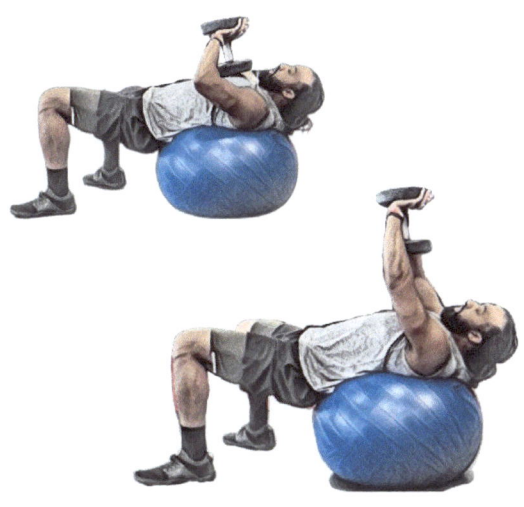

Barbell Bench Press

Lie down on a flat bench with your back fully pressed against it. Position your feet firmly on the ground, about shoulder-width apart. Grip the barbell slightly wider than shoulder-width apart, with your palms facing away. Lift the barbell off the rack and hold it directly above your chest with extended arms. Ensure that your wrists are straight and aligned with your forearms. Inhale and slowly lower the barbell towards your chest in a controlled manner. Keep your elbows at about a 45-degree angle to your body. Aim to lower the bar until it lightly touches your chest or hovers above it, depending on your flexibility and comfort level. Exhale and push the barbell to the starting position by extending your arms and contracting your chest muscles.

Keep your back flat on the bench throughout the movement and avoid arching excessively. Once you've completed your set, carefully rack the barbell back onto the rack. Ensure it's secure before releasing your grip.

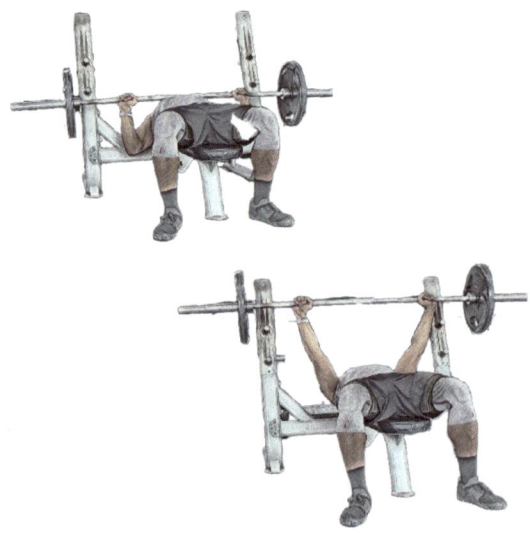

Alternating Barbell Bench Press

Lie down on a flat bench with your back fully pressed against it. Position your feet firmly on the ground, about shoulder-width apart. Grip the barbell slightly wider than shoulder-width apart, with your palms facing away. Lift the barbell off the rack and hold it directly above your chest with extended arms. Ensure that your wrists are straight and aligned with your forearms. Inhale and slowly lower one side of the barbell towards your chest in a controlled manner. Keep your elbow at about a 45-degree angle to your body. Aim to lower the bar until it lightly touches the outside of your chest or hovers just above it, depending on your flexibility and comfort level. Exhale and push the side of the barbell back up to the starting position by extending your arms and contracting your chest muscles. Keep your back flat on the bench throughout the movement and avoid arching excessively. Repeat on the opposite side. Once you've completed your set, carefully rack the barbell back onto the rack. Ensure it's secure before releasing your grip.

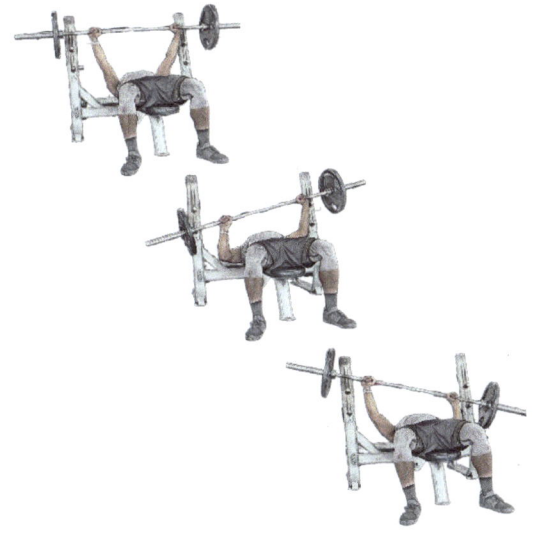

Clap Push Ups

Begin in a traditional push-up position with your hands slightly wider than shoulder-width apart, arms fully extended, and your body forming a straight line from your head to your heels. Engage your core and keep your back flat. Lower your body towards the ground by bending your elbows while keeping them close to your sides. Lower yourself until your chest nearly touches the floor, maintaining a controlled movement. Explosively push yourself back up by straightening your arms. As your arms fully extended, push off the ground with enough force to lift your hands off the ground. While in the air, quickly clap your hands together in front of your chest. As you descend back towards the ground, land with your hands in the starting position, ready to go into the next repetition.

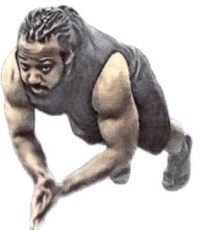

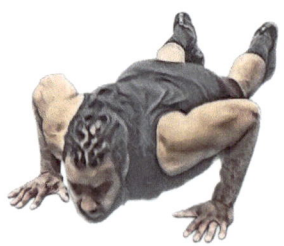

Superman Push Ups

Start in a traditional push-up position with your hands slightly wider than shoulder-width apart and your body in a straight line from head to heels.

Lower your chest towards the ground by bending your elbows, keeping them close to your body.

Once your chest is just above the ground, explosively push yourself up with enough force to lift both hands and feet off the ground simultaneously.

As you push off the ground, create enough momentum to allow your hands to move to the sides.

Quickly bring your hands back together underneath your shoulders and land softly, absorbing the impact with bent elbows.

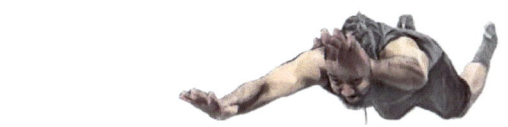

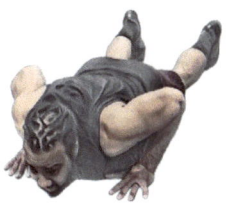

Plank Hops

Begin by placing a sturdy bench or elevated platform in front of you. Assume a plank position with your hands on the ground slightly wider than shoulder-width apart and your feet together or slightly apart for balance.

Engage your core muscles to keep your body straight from head to heels.

Lower your chest towards the ground by bending your elbows, keeping them close to your body.

As you push back up, explode with enough force to lift your hands off the ground.

Aim to land both hands simultaneously on the bench, ensuring a soft and controlled landing.

Once your hands are securely on the bench, lower yourself back into another push-up.

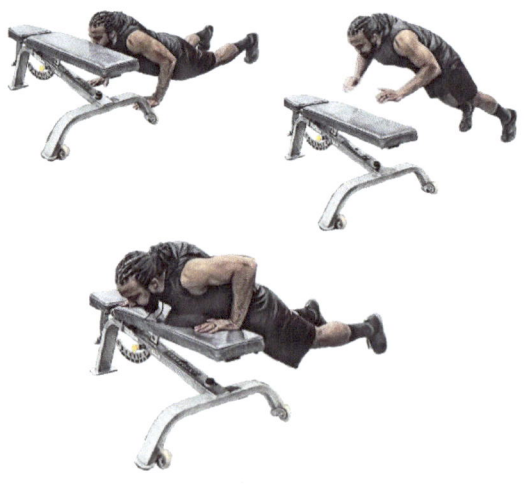

Plank Ups

Start in a plank position with your hands directly under your shoulders, arms fully extended, and your body forming a straight line from head to heels.

Engage your core muscles to stay stable and prevent your hips from sagging or sticking up.

Lower down onto your right forearm, followed by your left forearm, so you are now in a forearm plank position.

Push back onto your right hand, then your left hand, returning to the starting plank position.

Repeat this movement, alternating the arm you lower down onto first with each repetition.

Aim to keep your movements slow and controlled, focusing on maintaining proper form throughout

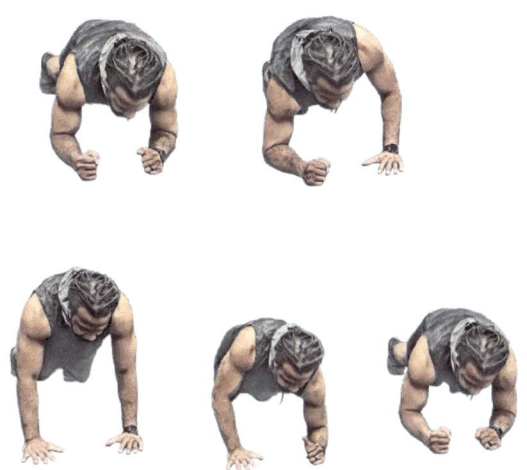

Plank Push Ups

Begin in an elbow plank position with your elbows directly under your shoulders and your body forming a straight line from head to heels. Engage your core muscles to maintain stability throughout the movement. Shift your weight forward slightly onto your toes, bringing your shoulders slightly past your elbows. Keep your body straight as you lower yourself towards the ground by bending your elbows, maintaining control and stability.

Lower your body until your chest is just above the ground or as low as you can comfortably go without letting your back arch or hips sag. Press through your palms and extend your elbows to push yourself back to the starting position.

Keep your core engaged and your body straighten throughout the movement.

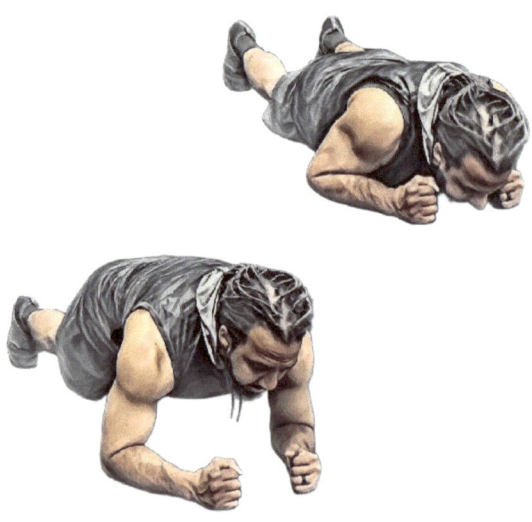

Stability Ball Push-ups

Start by placing the stability ball on the floor and positioning yourself facing down with your hands shoulder-width apart on the ball. Your feet should be extended behind you, balancing on your toes.

Engage your core muscles to maintain stability throughout the exercise. Lower your chest towards the ball by bending your elbows, keeping them close to your body. Your arms should form a 90-degree angle at the bottom of the movement.

Push yourself back up to the starting position by straightening your arms, but be mindful not to lock your elbows.

Always maintain proper form to avoid injury and maximize the effectiveness of the exercise.

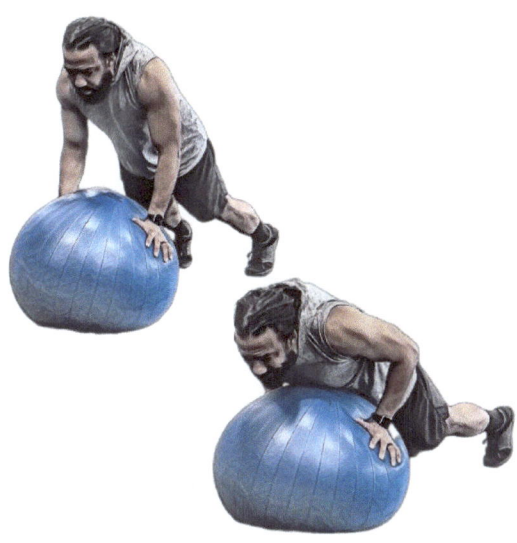

Resist Tube Chest Press on Stability Ball

Begin by sitting on a stability ball with your feet planted firmly on the ground, hip-width apart. Walk your feet forward as you roll down on the ball until the ball supports your head and upper back. Your knees should be at a 90-degree angle, and the ball should support your lower back. Grasp the ends of a resistance tube or band in each hand. The resistance level should be appropriate for your strength level and goals. Cross the resistance tube in front of you to create tension. Start with your arms extended straight up toward the ceiling, palms facing forward. Your elbows should be slightly bent. Exhale as you slowly lower your arms to the sides, keeping your elbows slightly bent. Lower until your elbows align with your shoulders or slightly below, feeling a stretch in your chest muscles. Inhale as you press the resistance tube handles back up to the starting position, bringing your hands close together without locking out your elbows. Throughout the exercise, maintain stability by engaging your core muscles and keeping your body aligned. Avoid excessive lower back arching or allowing the stability ball to roll.

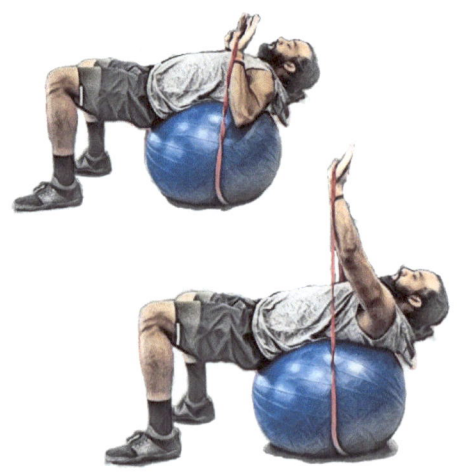

fasterstrongerwiser.com

Dumbbell Single Arm Chest Press on Stability Ball

Start by sitting on a stability ball with your feet planted firmly on the ground, hip-width apart. Hold a dumbbell in one hand and keep your core engaged to maintain balance. Slowly walk your feet forward as you roll down on the ball until your head and upper back are supported and your knees are bent at a 90-degree angle. The ball should support your lower back. Hold the dumbbell above your chest with your arm extended, palm facing away from you. Your elbow should be slightly bent. Inhale as you lower the dumbbell towards your chest in a controlled motion, keeping your elbow at a 90-degree angle. Exhale as you press the dumbbell back up to the starting position, fully extending your arm without locking your elbow. Repeat the desired repetitions on one arm before switching to the other. Remember to keep your core engaged throughout the exercise to maintain stability on the ball.

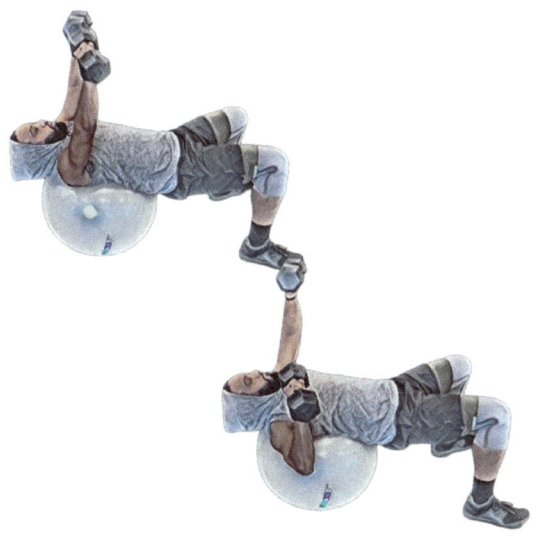

Resistance Band Pec Fly on Stability Ball

Set up your stability ball in an open space with enough room to move your arms freely. Place a resistance band around your wrists. Sit on the stability ball and carefully walk your feet forward until your upper back and head are comfortably resting on the ball. Your knees should be bent at a 90-degree angle, and your feet should be flat on the floor, hip-width apart, for stability. Extend your arms straight above your chest, shoulder-width apart. Engage your core muscles to stabilize your body on the stability ball. Slowly lower your arms to the sides in a controlled motion, keeping a slight bend in your elbows. Keep your hands in line with your shoulders as you lower your arms. Stop when your arms are parallel to the floor or feel a stretch in your chest muscles. Pause briefly, then slowly return to the starting position by squeezing your chest muscles and bringing your arms back together above your chest.

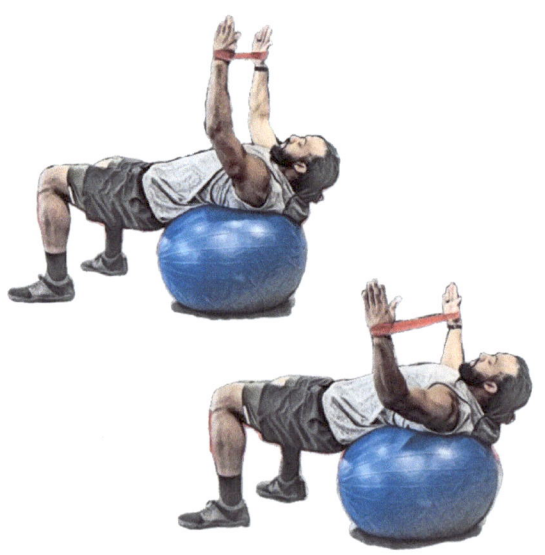

Thank You

I thank everyone for choosing and completing The Hectic Hundreds: Chest Workout Your commitment to your health and fitness journey is truly commendable, and I'm grateful that you chose this program to be a part of it.

I wish you all the best in your future endeavors, and may your path be filled with strength, vitality, and endless success.

With heartfelt thanks and warmest regards,

Glenn Payne,

Owner and Creator of Faster Stronger Wiser

www.ingramcontent.com/pod-product-compliance
Lightning Source LLC
Chambersburg PA
CBHW050838290526
45792CB00001B/448